CAREERS IN
VETERINARY MEDICINE

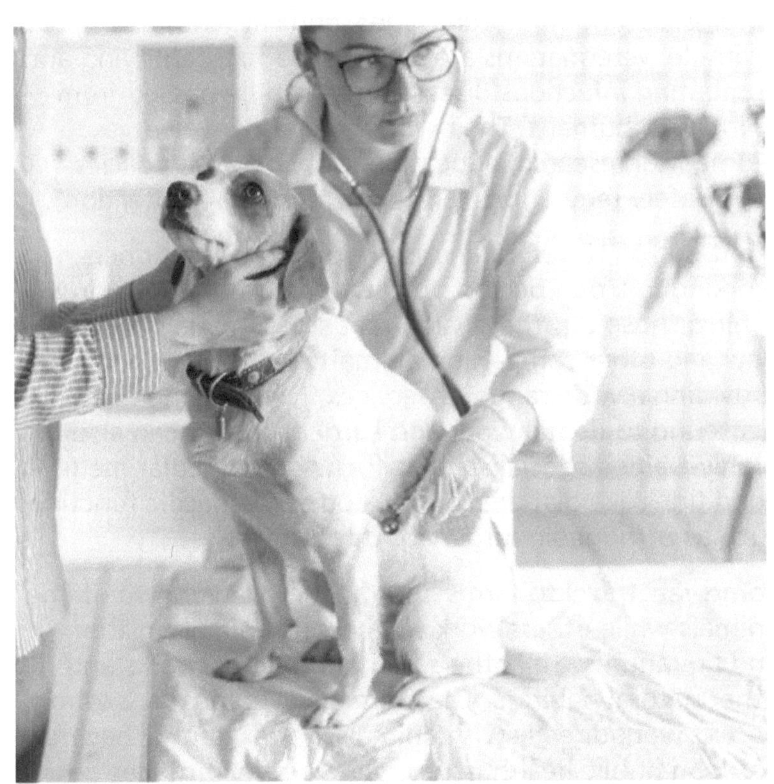

VETERINARIANS ARE DOCTORS WHO provide healthcare for animals. Like all doctors, they diagnose, treat, and research a wide variety of medical conditions using advanced procedures and sophisticated medical equipment. Their patients are often household pets, but they can also be livestock, zoo and aquarium dwellers, wildlife, or any other non-human animals.

Preventing disease and healing animals that are sick or injured are at the heart of what veterinarians do. The work is varied and activities go well beyond vaccinations, sutures, setting fractured bones, and surgeries. For example, veterinarians are responsible for identifying and combating infectious diseases that can be passed from animals to humans. Their work may also involve biomedical research, education, public health policies, food safety regulations, and environmental protection.

Eight out of 10 veterinarians are private practitioners, working in a one-person office or as part of a team in a clinic or hospital. These vets treat small animals, mostly pets and other companion animals. Most are generalists, providing a wide range of services from spaying and neutering to dental work and surgeries. They can also be highly-trained specialists that focus on particular medical conditions like diabetes or glaucoma, or specific functions such as orthopedic surgery or oncology.

Some vets travel to farms and ranches to work with large animals while others work with exotic animals in zoos and aquariums. Still others work in national parks and other natural habitats. There are also veterinarians who do not work directly with animals. For example, they may work on public health issues in government offices or conduct research in well-equipped laboratories.

Becoming a veterinarian is a lengthy process that takes at least eight years following high school graduation. To legally practice veterinary medicine, individuals are required to have a Doctor of Veterinary Medicine degree from an accredited veterinary college, as well as a state license. Vets who want to become board certified specialists will need to spend a few more years working in a clinical residency. When training is complete, the prospects of a new veterinarian finding employment are excellent. The demand for qualified veterinarians has never been stronger, especially for those with specialized skills.

Most vets report that their profession is quite rewarding. The pay is good with an average salary in the six figure range, and the opportunities are diverse and exciting. It can be challenging to deal with frightened animals who are sick or injured. It is sometimes equally difficult to interact with their owners who are also worried and stressed about their animals. For those with a passion for animals and great interpersonal skills, a career in veterinary medicine is an excellent career worth consideration.

WHAT YOU CAN DO NOW

IT IS NEVER TOO EARLY TO START PREPARING for a career as a veterinarian. Even a young teen in middle school can get a leg up by taking as many math and science classes as are available. A solid background in these subject areas will open up opportunities for college and beyond.

In high school, continue planning your curriculum around your future goals. Veterinary school admissions officers recommend a course load consisting of:

- Four years of math (calculus, algebra, geometry, & trigonometry)

- Four years of lab science (physics, biology, and chemistry)
- Four years of English

Getting into veterinary school is not easy. To be competitive, you will need to study hard and maintain a high GPA, and score high on SAT/ACT exams.

Extracurricular activities are important, too. Take part in after-school athletics, clubs, and groups that involve animals like 4-H and Future Farmers of America (FFA).

Because it takes years of rigorous training to become a veterinarian, you will want to make sure this is a good fit before you start down the path in this field. Find out what the work is really like by talking with real veterinarians. Most are happy to share stories of their own experiences, from what they did in high school up until they became established professionals. Be prepared to ask plenty of questions and get advice on how to best prepare. You can find vets to talk to simply by calling local veterinary offices or asking your guidance counselor to help you arrange a job shadow (or two).

Look for summer veterinary camps or other animal-centered programs for teens. These are often offered by colleges of veterinary medicine, but there are independent programs as well. For example, Global Leadership Adventures (GLA) provides international experiences that are similar to the usual vet camps, but are situated in other areas of the world. You might work on conservation efforts for elephants in Thailand or help improve the habitat for sea turtles in Costa Rica. Any enrichment activity you can add to your résumé will make your vet school application stand out.

Get as much experience with animals as possible. Get a part-time job, such as dog walking, pet sitting, dog grooming, cleaning horse stalls, working in a pet store, or helping out in a vet's office. If you cannot find a paying job, consider volunteering. Your local humane society or animal shelter can always use extra help. Local veterinarians, animal hospitals, and farms are other good possibilities for volunteer opportunities.

HISTORY OF THE PROFESSION

VETERINARY MEDICINE IN ANCIENT HISTORY followed a path similar to that of human medicine. Animals became domesticated around 8000 BC throughout the Middle East. Their importance in human life quickly grew as they became a primary food source. In the domestication process, disease ran rampant, and herdsmen had to care for the sick and keep the herds healthy. Their attempts at cures were primitive to say the least, consisting of magic, incantations, and other barbarous rituals. Knowledge of animal anatomy and diseases remained extremely limited for several thousand years.

The Egyptians were the first to make any meaningful advances. Egyptian hieroglyphs from 4000 BC depict using herbs to treat and promote good health in domesticated animals. A papyrus from around 1850 BC was the first known medical textbook that discussed animal anatomy. It also included instructions on how to spot certain diseases in a variety of animals and what specific treatments should be used to deal with them. Fast forward a thousand years, and the Romans, Greeks, Babylonians, Hindus, Arabs, and Hebrews were all practicing animal medicine, and researchers were using dissections to further their knowledge.

Attempts to organize those who were responsible for treating animals began in the Middle Ages. At that time, horses were of great economic importance. Farriers, who are basically horseshoers, were tasked with horse doctoring. The care horses received was poor, and it became clear that standards had to be established in order to improve animal care practices. In 1356, Lord Mayor of London initiated a fellowship among all farriers within a seven-mile radius of the city to regulate how they treated horses. The fellowship evolved into the Worshipful Company of Farriers in 1674.

Meanwhile, research continued. In 1598, the first comprehensive treatise on the anatomy of an animal species was published. Anatomia Del Cavallo (Anatomy of the Horse) was written by one of the earliest veterinary physicians, Carlo Ruini.

The Start of a Profession

Veterinary medicine became a recognized profession when the first veterinary school was founded in Lyon, France in 1761. Established by French veterinary surgeon Claude Bourgelat, the school was initially concerned with cattle plagues that had ravaged food animals throughout history. Students at the school learned the anatomy and diseases of sheep, horses, and cattle as well as instruction on how to apply vaccinations. Over the following 30 years, additional veterinary schools were established in Denmark, Germany, Sweden, and England. The initial focus of these schools continued to be horses and livestock, but dogs and other animals were eventually included.

The first professional association for veterinarians was formed in England in 1785. The stated purpose of the Odiham Agricultural Society was to encourage local industrial and agricultural development. It was resolved in its inaugural meeting that the Society should encourage and promote the study of farriery upon rational scientific principles. From that small tenet came the start of the deliberate development of veterinary science among professionals dedicated to animal medicine.

Veterinary Medicine in the United States

The first veterinary school established in the US was the Veterinary College of Philadelphia. It only operated from 1852 to 1866. In 1883, the oldest accredited veterinary school still in operation today was opened at the University of Pennsylvania. Other veterinary schools were soon opened in Boston and New York. In 1879, the Iowa Agricultural College became the first land grant college to offer veterinary medicine programs.

Around this same time in the late 19th century, the American Veterinary Medical Association (AVMA) was established, and the Bureau of Animal Industry was organized under the USDA. The Bureau did not last long, but while in operation its objective was important and transformative: to protect the public from infectious diseases through contaminated meat, eradicate diseases in animals and improve the quality of livestock.

20th Century Veterinarians

Following the invention of the internal combustion engine in the early 1900s, the need of animals for transportation and farming declined drastically. Veterinarians who had previously focused on those big animals had to make adjustments to survive. They did so by including the treatment of dogs and cats into their business. Small animal work soon became a field of its own.

As World War I came to an end, new fields in veterinary medicine opened up. For example, poultry had become one of the most important industries in the US. Some small animal medical practitioners learned how to work with poultry species, such as chickens, turkeys, and ducks. By specializing in poultry medicine, these experts were able to build thriving businesses.

Throughout the first few decades of the 20th century, notable achievements were made in veterinary research, systems of education, and the development of improved equipment and medicines. Terrible diseases like bovine tuberculosis were eradicated, and advances in parasitology conquered a host of parasites that had been around for millennia.

Throughout the second half of the century, the AVMA and other professional veterinary groups advocated for the veterinarian as a medical professional, to be considered equal to human doctors.

By the 1950s, dogs and cats were occupying more than half of American households. At the same time, more people lived in cities and suburbs than in rural farming areas. As a result, pets became the primary patients for most veterinarians.

Veterinary medicine has now evolved from a traveling farrier tending to farmer's horses and cows, to highly trained and licensed physicians with gleaming exam rooms and digital equipment. Gone are the old poultices, tinctures, and other crude topicals meant to heal. Now we have a vast array of anesthetics, chemotherapeutic drugs, vaccinations, pain relievers, and treatments for every imaginable malady.

Today's veterinarians are on the cutting edge of medicine, able to diagnose medical problems with ultrasound and endoscopy. They can also run complete blood panels in minutes, perform a variety of surgical procedures with effective pain management, transplant organs, do bone grafts, replace hips and other bones, and generally keep animals alive and healthy much longer than nature might have intended.

WHERE YOU WILL WORK

THERE ARE ABOUT 85,000 VETERINARIANS working in the US today. The vast majority of those – about four out of five – work in private practice, providing healthcare for pets and other companion animals. Yet there are thousands of other opportunities for employment outside the small animal clinic setting.

Some veterinarians work for corporations that provide animal care services or animal-related products, such as big box pet stores, pet food companies, food processing plants, and pharmaceutical manufacturers. Many others work on farms and ranches, in animal shelters, zoos and aquariums, or at race tracks. Those with high-level training are employed to conduct research in private laboratories, at universities, or for various government agencies. A small number work in national parks and other natural habitat settings.

There are also a surprising number of jobs that have veterinarians working in an office setting. Some are specialists who provide consulting services, while others are involved in advocacy roles or provide services that are closely related to veterinary practices, such as agricultural management.

In addition to the many jobs within industry and academia, there are veterinarians working at all levels of government in the fields of public health or regulatory medicine. All states, and many counties and cities, depend on veterinarians to help control animal diseases. The federal government, through its many agencies, employs far more veterinarians than state and local governments combined. The single biggest government employer of veterinarians is the US Department of Agriculture, followed by the National Institutes of Health

(NIH) and the Centers for Disease Control (CDC). Veterinarians working in these agencies are primarily concerned with public health, and work to prevent and control animal-borne diseases that are transmissible to humans. They inspect milk, meats, and other food products of animal origin to ensure they are safe to consume, and investigate any food-borne disease outbreaks. They are also responsible for overseeing the interstate transport of animals.

There are also veterinarians in the US Air Force and US Army. Some provide care for government-owned animals, while others inspect food or serve as biomedical research investigators.

Work Environment

The most common setting for veterinary work is the animal clinic or hospital. These facilities are usually well lit and clean, but are also filled with activity and noise. Those working in research spend their days in immaculate laboratories, while those working on policy may do their work in an office.

Veterinarians who care for large animals typically spend most of their time outside. They may work in zoos, on farms and ranches, or with wildlife in remote locations. These professionals are subjected to all kinds of weather, even while performing difficult procedures such as surgery or obstetrics.

Travel for most vets is limited to local visits to farms, slaughterhouses, and food processing plants. However, there is a growing number of vets who are choosing to make life more convenient and less stressful for pets and their owners by operating out of well-equipped mobile clinics.

Work Schedule

The standard operating hours for veterinarians in private practice are the usual 9am to 6pm during the week. However, the hours can actually end up being quite lengthy depending on the type and location of the practice. It is common for vets to be on call for emergencies after hours and on weekends, especially in locations where there are fewer vets to rely on. In some instances, such as animal hospitals that offer emergency services, overnight shifts may be required.

THE WORK YOU WILL DO

A VETERINARIAN IS A DOCTOR WHO SPECIALIZES in the treatment of animals. Just like human doctors, they diagnose, treat, and research medical conditions and diseases. However, their patients are pets, livestock, wildlife, zoo denizens, and other animals.

Likewise, veterinarians use a variety of medical equipment that is very similar to that used by human physicians, like aspirators, digital x-ray and ultrasound machines, catheters, pin drivers, and surgical tools. They also use equipment that is designed specifically for animal care, such as specialty scales, anesthesia systems, insemination equipment, and sonic micro-fissure detection tools.

Despite the similarities, there are major differences between human medicine and veterinary medicine. A medical doctor only treats humans. A veterinarian is trained to treat a wide array of animal species. A human doctor can (usually) ask the patient where it hurts, while animals cannot verbalize their condition. In human medicine, nearly every type of health issue or treatment is compartmentalized. For example, cancer cases or functions such as surgery or anesthesia must be referred to specialists in those disciplines. Veterinarians can refer complicated cases to specialists, but they do not have to. They can perform most procedures on their own.

In addition to caring for the health of animals, veterinarians are at the forefront of protecting the public's health and well-being. They conduct research that promotes the health and safety of both animals and humans. They work to identify and control the spread of diseases within animal populations and also those that are transmittable to humans. They make sure the nation's food supply is safe.

Animals Big and Small

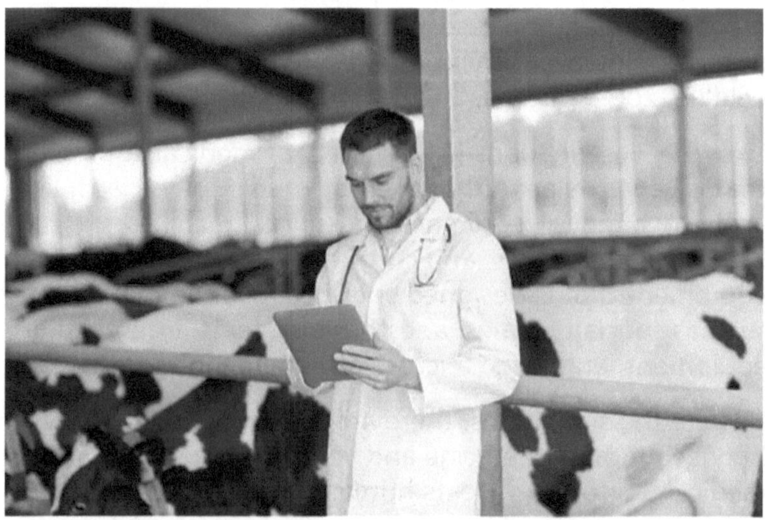

There are more than a million animal species in the world and no veterinarian is going to treat them all. Veterinarians generally work with animals in one of three categories: small, large, and exotic. Small animal vets are the most common. These professionals work mostly with dogs and cats, but will also care for virtually any kind of companion animals like hamsters, guinea pigs, birds, reptiles, rodents, and fish, that people might keep as pets. Some small animal vets receive extra training to deal with some of the more exotic small animal species.

Large animal vets work primarily on farms and ranches, which means they spend a significant amount of time traveling to different locations. Most of these professionals are food animal veterinarians who specialize in treating meat producing animals like sheep, goats, pigs, fowl, and cattle. Their duties include treating sick and injured animals, testing for diseases common to herd animals, implementing preventive measures like giving shots and vaccinations, and ensuring that the animals are in a healthy environment. They also provide advice about feeding, housing, and other general health issues. Unlike small animal vets, these practitioners may also be involved in livestock breeding.

There are also large animal veterinarians who devote their attention to working animals, such as those in the equine industry. Horses have a long history of working for humans. For thousands of years, they have been used for transport, hunting, warfare, and agriculture. Today, their jobs are fewer, including mostly racing, police work, ranching, and entertainment.

Large animal vets are often generalists, but specializations are common. For example, there are equine veterinarians that work with racehorses. They spend their days at racetracks and horse training facilities, ensuring horses stay healthy, collecting samples for drug testing and tending to injuries.

Exotic animal vets are usually found at zoos and aquariums, caring for everything from alligators to zebras. A few have private practices that are dedicated to exotic pets like snakes, monkeys, and tropical birds. Keeping captive animals healthy requires constant vigilance. A wild animal's survival instincts often prevent them from displaying any obvious symptoms since any sign of weakness would make them vulnerable to predators. Therefore, the best veterinarians for this environment are those with exceptional observation skills. In addition to keeping animals in good shape, zoo and aquarium vets help replicate natural habitats and are often heavily involved in conservation activities and public education.

There are also exotic animal vets working in natural habitat settings, in national parks, and other wild and open areas. These vets help rehabilitate injured animals, protect animal populations, and work to prevent and control disease within certain species. They work to ensure that animals have a healthy environment in which they can thrive, whether it is a desert, rain forest, or ocean. Unlike private practitioners, these are specialists who work almost exclusively outdoors.

Private Practice

The vast majority of veterinarians – about 80 percent – work in private practice, caring for companion animals. This can be a one-person vet office or a larger facility, such as an animal clinic or hospital. Private practices of any size can offer services that are relatively general or incredibly specific.

Private practitioners offer many different services. What they do will depend on the particular practice, but the following are the most common routine tasks in a general practice.

- Conduct well-pet and other exams to assess general health

- Offer preventive healthcare, like testing for and vaccinating against parasites and diseases

- Diagnose and treat medical problems like infections, abscesses, and kidney failure

- Provide emergency care

- Dress wounds and set broken bones

- Spay and neuter

- Perform surgical procedures and dental work

- Prescribe medication

- Euthanize animals

Private practice vets also interact with animal owners. They provide advice about preventive healthcare, nutrition, reproductive issues, the need for euthanasia, behavioral problems, or other issues that can affect an animal's well-being. They also provide instructions on how to manage medical conditions, administer medications, or clean and dress wounds.

Most veterinarians in private practice are generalists, capable of handling a wide range of services. However, there are many situations that would benefit from calling in a specialist. For example, if a dog is genetically susceptible to certain conditions like glaucoma or hip dysplasia, an animal ophthalmologist or orthopedic surgeon could offer valuable experience and skills that a generalist might not possess.

Specializations

Just like human doctors, veterinarians can choose to become specialists. This sometimes means focusing on a particular type of animal, but more often it means having the additional training and board certification to offer specialty services. There are a number of specialties to choose from, including:

- Anesthesia
- Animal behavior
- Cardiology
- Dentistry
- Dermatology
- Emergency and critical care
- Internal medicine
- Neurology
- Oncology
- Orthopedics
- Radiology

Veterinary specialists typically have their own practices, offering consulting services to those in general practice.

Roles Beyond Private Practice

Veterinarians do not necessarily have to work directly with animals, providing treatment and other medical procedures in clinical settings. Many work in offices, laboratories, and classrooms, rather than at pet hospitals, zoos, or farms. For example, some veterinarians work part time or full time as consultants to various businesses and organizations. They might be on retainer or hired on an ad hoc basis when their expertise is needed by humane societies, 4-H, dairy farmers, animal rights advocates, or legislators.

Public health and regulatory medicine are other fields for office-based veterinarians. These professionals understand that human health is often dependent on animal health. They are found throughout government, employed by every state in the US, as well as many counties and cities. As public health officials, they play critical roles in environmental protection, food and water safety, disease control, and even homeland security.

Those in regulatory medicine are hired to inspect meat and dairy products, test for livestock disease, and oversee the interstate transport of animals. Some design and administer new animal and public health programs to control diseases, while others are hired to enforce existing government food safety regulations.

Food safety is of major concern to public health veterinarians. Those who specialize in this important role work to ensure millions of Americans can eat meat, poultry, dairy products, eggs, and other animal products without fear of falling ill. They are responsible for continually inspecting these products, testing livestock for outbreaks of disease that could potentially jump from animals to humans, providing vaccines to prevent outbreaks, and conducting epidemiological research that could lead to new ways to protect the public from food-borne illnesses. They also develop and test new farm control methods to detect and prevent the spread of dangerous contaminants like salmonella, E coli or other pathogens.

While many food safety specialists work in offices or laboratories, some do work in other settings along the food supply chain. This includes food processing plants. The primary concern of these veterinarians is making sure animals are treated humanely. They also enforce regulations, test for drug residues, and evaluate facility conditions.

Veterinarians also work in laboratories. Some have advanced training in pathology or microbiology and specialize in diagnostics. Diagnostics laboratories might hire them to utilize state of the art equipment to analyze samples of tissue or blood and make accurate diagnoses for veterinary medical practices that do not have such elaborate setups. These laboratories are often affiliated with medical teaching hospitals, but they may also be privately owned and operated by small firms or large corporations.

Some veterinarians working in laboratories are involved in biomedical research, which is a rapidly growing field. Specialists in this area are hired by pharmaceutical and private research laboratories, universities, and various government agencies to advance the fields of toxicology and microbiology as they relate to animal and human health. The most common research projects involve developing and testing new vaccines, serums, and other biological agents that could treat and control diseases in both animals and humans. There are also molecular biologists researching immunity, genetics, longevity, and the nature of specific diseases.

Laboratory research sometimes involves working with lab animals. Laboratory animal veterinarians are specialists who oversee the housing, feeding, breeding, and general health of animals used in research. While conducting research, they are also responsible for providing regular veterinary care for the animals and monitoring disease control programs.

There are also thousands of veterinarians teaching on university campuses, in medical schools, agricultural schools, and veterinary schools.

VETS TELL THEIR OWN STORIES

I Am a General Practitioner

"Veterinary medicine is an amazing field. When you love animals as much as I (and most other veterinarians) do, your desire to help them grows stronger every day. I highly recommend considering this career path, but it is important to get a realistic picture of what to expect. Every job has its pros and cons, and veterinary medicine is no different.

Many people think vets just play with kittens and puppies all day. While there is a high level of cuteness involved, this work is anything but play. Even when I don't work late, I am often exhausted by the time I get home. Appointments are nonstop and there is always an emergency to squeeze in somehow.

Cute or not, animals can be difficult to handle because they are terrified. The vet's office is an unfamiliar environment, with sounds of other wounded and scared animals, and strange people doing things to them that they don't understand. I do everything I can to minimize their fear, but I've been scratched and bitten more times than I can count.

Vets don't spend all their time working with animals either. A big part of the job is working with people and that isn't always easy. How do you explain that their beloved pet should be euthanized? Or why their expensive vet bill is justified? They may not have realistic expectations for what I can do or understand that vet training is just as rigorous as med school. It can take a long time to figure out how to communicate effectively to my patients' owners.

What it all adds up to is a career that I absolutely love. I get to spend my days relieving the suffering of sick and injured animals and preventing problems in those that are healthy. Occasionally, I will get to share the excitement of a child with a new pet. Doing what you love makes a world of difference in how you feel about your career."

I Am an Animal Eye Doctor

"As an animal eye specialist, I can perform a long list of procedures. I routinely do microsurgery, corneal grafts, retinal repairs, and cataract surgery. It is surprising how many eye ailments in people are shared by animals of all kinds. Some conditions are inherited among high-risk breeds like glaucoma in cocker spaniels and poodles. Others are caused by infections or metabolic disorders like diabetes. Then there are trauma cases resulting from collisions with vehicles, cat spats, or owners letting their dogs stick their heads out the car window.

I see mostly dogs in my practice, but like most veterinary ophthalmologists, I will treat any creature with an eye. Although about one in 10 veterinary visits involves eye problems, there are fewer than a thousand eye specialists in the US. That is not nearly enough to keep up with the demand. I keep very busy caring for pets, but am also called in on cases in zoos and aquariums around the state. So far, my 'special' patients have included gorillas, walruses, kangaroos, flying foxes, and Beluga whales.

It takes a lot of training to be qualified to practice any of the many specialty disciplines in veterinary medicine. Unlike general practitioners who spend eight years going to college and then vet school, I also had to do an internship for a year and three more years of residency after graduation.

It was grueling, but worth every bleary-eyed moment. I get to work on the cutting edge of veterinary medicine, putting new developments in gene therapy to work and helping pioneer new treatments in inherited disorders that can cause blindness in both puppies and young children. I do it because I love working with animals, and I have a lot of cool tools to play with."

PERSONAL QUALIFICATIONS

MOST, IF NOT ALL, PEOPLE WHO PURSUE a career in veterinary medicine do so because they love animals. Their passion for animals often started in childhood with a beloved family pet or excited visits to the zoo or aquarium. Some grew up on farms or ranches. Whatever sparked their inspiration, veterinary medicine seemed the obvious career choice. The veterinary profession is a diverse occupation that is challenging from the moment one starts preparing for the lengthy, difficult training until you are working on your own, facing challenging situations on a daily basis.

Many veterinarians have managed to climb the career ladder with hard work, commitment, and a great deal of knowledge. The most successful have the advantage of possessing certain personality and physical traits that are ideally suited for the work of a veterinarian. Take a look at these characteristics and see if you have them.

Successful veterinarians have a deep sense of compassion for their patients. It is what drives them to provide the best care they possibly can. They have a unique ability to communicate that empathy to their patients, calming and comforting them while working on diagnosing and solving their medical problems. This is an innate skill that schools cannot really teach. This compassion also extends to the animal owners who may be scared and worried about the pets that are often considered family members.

It is important to treat animal owners with sensitivity and respect. This is not always as simple as it sounds. Some vets enter the profession with the belief that they will be dealing only with animals, not people. In fact, it is common for veterinarians to be introverts, which is not a helpful characteristic. Owners from pet parents to farm owners can be difficult to deal with. Some may be unpleasant or upset about the cost of care. Others may be irrational and expect unreasonable outcomes. It will take exceptional interpersonal and communications skills to handle the range of people attached to your patients.

The work of a veterinarian can be physically demanding. How much strength and stamina are needed will depend on the particular job situation. Muscle power is needed to lift and restrain large animals, whether it is on a farm, at a zoo, or in the wild. Even smaller animals seem to acquire super strength when they are hurt and scared. You have to be quick and equally strong to avoid their biting, kicking, and scratching. Manual dexterity is needed to perform precision surgeries and other tricky procedures. Stamina is needed to work long hours, especially when animals need help throughout the night.

Strong problem-solving skills are essential. Figuring out what is wrong with an animal is not always easy, but it is necessary to determine the appropriate treatment.

Decisions also need to be made quickly, especially in emergency cases when any delay could mean failure.

A head for business is a big plus in this field. Many veterinarians are in private practice, with responsibilities that range from hiring and managing staff to making sure revenues outpace expenses. Being a great entrepreneur with sharp business skills is an intrinsic characteristic that successful veterinarians have in common. Basic business skills can be learned though. Veterinary students should determine early on if owning a business is their goal. If so, enrolling in marketing, accounting, and other business courses would be advisable.

ATTRACTIVE FEATURES

THE VETERINARY PROFESSION IS ONE of the most interesting and diverse careers there is. What is it really like to be a veterinarian? Some days it can be difficult, stressful, and sad. Other days are filled with success and happiness. Overall, it is rewarding and fulfilling to work with your passion and make animals feel better. There are a number of other attractive features that come with this career.

Obviously, becoming a veterinarian gives you the chance to help animals. This is probably the number one most rewarding part of the job. However, in the process you also get to help people. Families often regard their pets as members of the family, which comes with deep emotional attachments. There is tremendous satisfaction in helping families save their pets who are in bad condition get on the road to recovery. In times of difficulty, they serve as counselors to owners who have to make the difficult decisions like whether to euthanize an animal.

In addition to helping individuals, veterinarians also make important contributions to human health in the community. They play critical roles in food safety, environmental protection, and public health. Veterinarians are the ones who made discoveries that helped control malaria and yellow fever, solved the mystery of botulism, produced an anticoagulant to treat heart disease, and found the cause of West Nile virus. They also developed permanent artificial limbs and new treatments for broken bones and joint disease. All of these accomplishments started with helping animals, but evolved into major advances in medicine for humans.

Veterinarians earn good money. Even starting salaries are above average at more than $50,000. With experience there is an opportunity to earn well into six figures. Those who obtain training and board certification in high-demand areas of specializations can earn as much as $350,000. There is also the potential to increase earnings by opening a clinic rather than depending on a salary from someone else. However, that requires some business acumen and the nerve to be self-reliant.

There are plenty of good jobs available for veterinarians, and the job outlook for the foreseeable future is excellent. Over the next 10 years, the number of positions available for veterinarians is expected to grow by almost 20 percent, which is well above the average for other occupations. The demand for good vets is growing because people are more willing than ever to pay for a high level of care for their animals. It is an excellent time for someone to pursue a degree in veterinary medicine.

Veterinarians enjoy a wide range of diverse opportunities. Vets can work with animals of every description, large and small, whether in zoos, farms and ranches, or pet clinics. They can specialize in specific areas of veterinary medicine, such as radiology, dentistry, critical care, or ophthalmology. They can also utilize their training and be a surgeon, anesthesiologist, and obstetrician all at once. A degree in veterinary medicine is also applicable to different industry applications. While most vets work in private practice, opportunities exist to work in research, education, diagnostic laboratories, consultation, pharmaceutical manufacturing, and public health and regulatory medicine.

UNATTRACTIVE ASPECTS

BEING SURROUNDED BY ADORABLE ANIMALS every day certainly has its appeal. That is just one of the benefits of working as a veterinarian. Like any career, it also has its downsides. Before taking the plunge, consider both pros and cons carefully.

Veterinarians are at risk for injuries and illnesses. Animals that are in pain and scared instinctively lash out because they do not necessarily understand that you are trying to help them. It is common for vets to be bitten, scratched, and kicked when working with hurt animals. There is also the possibility of being infected by the disease of the animals you are working with. Most serious problems are prevented by getting anti-rabies shots and other vaccines.

The work can be emotionally stressful. Part of the job is euthanizing animals to relieve unnecessary suffering, caring for abused animals, and providing support to anxious and overwrought owners. Some veterinarians also succumb to compassion fatigue. It is estimated that veterinarians experience death of patients five times more often than human doctors. That can take its toll. After some time in the field, veterinarians can get emotionally drained and lose their ability to recover from such experiences. When they start to feel numb to both patients and their home life, they often have no choice but to leave the profession.

Getting started in this career is not easy. It takes eight years of training and anywhere from $35,000 to $50,000 per year in tuition and fees. Just gaining admission to one of the 30 accredited vet schools is a rigorous process. Once admitted, the real work begins. Vet school courses are challenging because they are very technical. It could even be argued that vet school is tougher than med school because medical doctors only have to learn about humans while vets have to know more than one species.

Treating sick animals is a messy business. Animals are brought into clinics because they are sick, and some might soon die. Treating a wounded animal requires fortitude and a high tolerance for blood, vomit, urine, parasites, and other unpleasantries.

Veterinarians can find themselves being overworked. Due to the shortage of vets, there may be no backup to call on when an animal needs help after the regular workday has ended. Overtime is not unusual, and many vets are on call nights and weekends. This can make it hard to balance your work and family life. It can also create constant fatigue.

EDUCATION AND TRAINING

THE PATH TO BECOMING A VETERINARIAN is long and difficult. In order to practice, all veterinarians must have a Doctor of Veterinary Medicine degree from an accredited veterinary college, as well as a state license. This typically takes at least eight years following high school graduation to achieve. Most applicants to veterinary medical school have a bachelor's degree, but it is not always required for entrance. However, a significant number of credit hours amounting to at least three years of study at the undergraduate level are required of everyone.

Arguably, the hardest part is getting into veterinary medical school. There are only 30 accredited colleges of veterinary medicine (CVMs) in the US, which is not nearly enough to accommodate the number of aspiring vets. How many applicants manage to get in depends on the size of the applicant pool and how many positions are offered, but it is estimated that the average acceptance rate is about 10 to 15 percent. Therefore, it is necessary to start preparing and finding ways to maximize your chance for acceptance as early as possible.

Ideally, college undergraduates would take a pre-vet or comparable curriculum, but it is not absolutely necessary. According to the Association of American Veterinary Medical Colleges (AAVMC), veterinary medical students come from all kinds of backgrounds and majors, including the arts or humanities. What is important is that any curriculum includes the prerequisite math and science courses like biology and chemistry.

Regardless of the major, mediocre grades will not suffice. Applicants are expected to maintain a high GPA. If a candidate's grades are not high, chances of getting accepted by any veterinary medical school is minimal. Students would also benefit from joining a pre-vet club.

It is important to gain practical experience with veterinary medicine right away. This could start with job shadowing veterinarians and animal research scientists, or possibly working on a farm. Most experts recommend getting at least four years of practical experience to increase the chances of vet school acceptance. You can do this while you are in high school. The surest way to manage this is to look for opportunities to volunteer. The most likely places to volunteer include local vet clinics, veterinarian hospitals, or animal shelters. Be careful to avoid being pigeonholed into any one type of veterinary work. There are many different types of jobs and the broader your exposure, the better. Look for opportunities to work with exotic animals in zoos, horses at racetracks or stables, or wildlife in their natural habitat.

Veterinarian School

Once in veterinary school, students will study veterinary medicine for a minimum of four years. Coursework for the first three years will cover animal anatomy, physiology, disease prevention, diagnosis, and treatment. Subjects will be taught through classroom instruction and laboratory work. Students will have the opportunity to decide which specific field they want to focus on, such as domestic animals, reptiles and birds, or marine life. The final year of a four-year program will involve a clinical component, which usually means doing clinical rotations in a veterinary medical center or hospital.

Many veterinary students continue training in order to specialize in disciplines such as cardiology, dermatology, internal medicine, oncology, ophthalmology, radiology, or surgery. This additional high-level training takes about two years on average.

Licenses and Certifications

Veterinarians must be licensed in order to practice in the United States. At the national level, all prospective veterinarians must complete an accredited veterinary program and pass the North American Veterinary Licensing Examination. State licensing requirements vary, but most states also require veterinarians to pass a state licensing exam. State exams generally cover that particular state's laws and regulations regarding animal medicine. To legally practice in more than one state, veterinarians would need to take additional exams for the states where they want to be licensed. In some cases, veterinarians may not need a state license. There are sometimes exceptions for those employed by state or federal government agencies, and in the military.

In most cases, certification is not necessary to practice veterinary medicine. Certifications are available for those who have moved beyond performing broad-based clinical practice and demonstrated they have the training and capability of providing superior veterinary care in a specialized discipline. The American Board of Veterinary Practitioners (ABVP) is the recognized specialty organization that offers board certifications in 11 veterinary specialties.

Continuing Education

The field of veterinary medicine is constantly changing, and it is important for all vets to learn and practice with the latest knowledge. For this reason, continuing education courses and additional exams are often required to maintain a veterinarian's license.

EARNINGS

VETERINARIANS ON AVERAGE EARN ABOUT $95,000 A year. Most earn between $70,000 and $125,000, but the overall range is significantly wider. The lowest 10 percent earn less than $60,000, and the highest 10 percent earn more than $165,000. Differences in pay depend on geographic location, area of specialization, and certification.

This is the base pay. Most vets also earn various forms of additional cash compensation that amounts to an average of more than $10,000. Again, there is a wide range. The average yearly bonus is roughly $5,000, but can be as much as $20,000. Commissions are also common. They can add more than $40,000 to a vet's yearly pay, but the average is more like $15,000. Profit sharing is less common, but those lucky vets who benefit from the arrangement take home an average of $10,000 per year.

States where veterinarians are paid the most include New York, Massachusetts, and Maryland where the salaries are routinely well into the six figure range. Most other states have vets earning in the high $80,000s and $90,000s. The lowest paying states are in the South and Midwest, including North Carolina, Mississippi, Florida, Missouri, Michigan, and Illinois.

The highest earnings are claimed by veterinarians who practice within certain specialty areas. Specialties like lab animal medicine, ophthalmology, pathology, surgery, internal medicine, radiology, and theriogenology (reproduction) all pay more than $200,000 a year. The rewards for the very best specialists (those in the 90th percentile) are even more impressive. Top ophthalmologists and radiologists earn more than

$300,000 per year. The best pathologists, surgeons and lab animal medicine specialists also do quite well at more than $250,000 a year.

Board certification can also make a big difference in earnings. Across all categories, veterinarians without board certification earn significantly less than those with board certification. Even top specialists without board certification only earn about half of what similarly accomplished certified vets earn. The disparity continues throughout non-specialty areas. Private practice and corporate veterinarians in government or industry without board certification earn a median income of $90,000 per year. That is a bit lower than the national average overall. By contrast, board certification for those professionals can bring their median income up to a respectable $185,000. The main reason for this difference is the severe shortage of board certified specialists.

While the potential financial rewards are certainly attractive, it should be noted that care for animals is typically considered discretionary. In good economic times, pet owners and even farm owners are able and willing to pay for treatments. However, when the economy dips, there is a natural tendency to save money by delaying healthcare. Unfortunately, this is often short-sighted since bringing animals to a vet at a later stage when conditions have deteriorated can mean more expensive treatments or it may even be too late.

OPPORTUNITIES

THIS IS AN EXCELLENT TIME FOR SOMEONE to pursue a career in veterinary medicine. The outlook for veterinarian employment is positive, and it will only improve in the future. The number of positions for veterinarians is projected to grow by almost 20 percent over the coming decade. That is well above the average for other occupations. Industry surveys concur. Various surveys indicate that there will be a steadily increasing demand for veterinary medical doctors and scientists in the future.

The main reason behind the rosy job outlook is a general change in attitude among pet owners. In the past, people often avoided taking their pets to a veterinarian because they saw it as a voluntary, unnecessary expense. That has changed. Today, people are spending more money than ever on their pets, for everything from gourmet pet food to doggie daycare. In fact, a staggering $75 billion is now being spent each year on American pets, and a good portion of that is going toward high-level healthcare. Veterinary medicine has advanced considerably, to the point it is often comparable to healthcare for humans with services ranging from vaccinations to complicated cancer treatments and kidney transplants.

While the demand for services is increasing, the ability to gain admission to the limited number of training programs is not. There is a shortfall of qualified new vets to fill the many jobs that are available. Especially urgent is the need for those who are trained and board certified in specialty areas.

The majority of veterinarians will continue to work in private clinical practice, handling small companion animals. However, the types of animals in need of veterinary services have become an important issue. The demand for vets who can work with larger animals is increasing because fewer vets are choosing to treat bigger animals. Rural areas in particular are in dire need of veterinary professionals to treat horses, bulls, and cows.

The public's concern for animal welfare and biomedical/environmental research is also driving demand. Veterinary medicine is heavily involved in issues of food quality, human health, energy, and environmental quality. There is a present demand for veterinary specialists who deal with food animals as well as research veterinarians who can deal with society's interests in these other issues. Research jobs are constantly opening up in pharmaceutical and private research laboratories, universities, and various government agencies.

The greatest number of job opportunities will continue to exist in California, Texas, Florida, and New York. The fewest are in small states like Rhode Island and Delaware and sparsely populated states like Alaska and North Dakota.

GETTING STARTED

AFTER SO MUCH HARD WORK, IT IS EXCITING to finally be a fully trained and licensed veterinarian. Now it is time to look for your very first veterinary job. Many graduates start by completing one-year internships to gain real working experience and improve their skills. Internships can also transition into full-time jobs. The American Association of Veterinary Clinicians (AAVC) sponsors an internship and residency program that matches interns with participating private practices. Internships are also posted on job sites.

If you have already completed an internship, check out your school's career center. Visit the center often. New job listings will be posted as they come up and there will be notices of recruiters scheduled to visit. There are other valuable services, too. For example, creating a strong résumé and cover letter may not be in your skillset. At the career center, you can get help writing a résumé that will stand out to potential employers, and will also help you practice your interviewing techniques.

Next, move your search online. Any of the major online job sites like ZipRecruiter and Indeed will have thousands of veterinarian job openings posted. At the moment, ZipRecruiter alone has more than 35,000! You can use the various search fields to hone in on exactly what you are looking for, including location, job duties, hours, full time or part time, and salary. Your best bet is to look for Associate Veterinarian positions.

Most of the listings on the job sites are private practices or corporate employers that deal with small animals. If your goal is to work in a zoo, aquarium, or research facility, you will need to look elsewhere. The best source of opportunities is professional trade publications, such as Zoo News Digest.

Many of the best veterinary positions are filled from the inside without ever being advertised or listed on a job board. You can seek them out the old school way by compiling a list of animal clinics, pet hospitals, and other facilities in the area where you want to work and start calling or emailing.

There is an even better way. Start networking – immediately. Networking is your most powerful job search tool. The best way to learn about upcoming job openings is to talk with people who may be in a position to know about them. You should have a collection of contacts starting with all your teachers and professors. Supervisors from internships, volunteer work, and paid jobs are particularly useful resources when searching for the right job after you graduate. Professional organizations are also very good for forming networking connections that could lead to career opportunities. Join, mingle, and actively participate in workshops, seminars, and other activities where members get together. Even small meetings provide a special opportunity to interact with established professionals who may know someone who is hiring.

Once you get called for an interview, do your homework and research the employer. The facility's website and corresponding online reviews should provide all the relevant information you need. Be prepared to describe the business, point out what appeals to you, and why you think you would be a good fit. Feel free to ask for a tour of the facility and be ready to ask your own questions. Show you are interested in working there and they will be more interested in working with you.

ASSOCIATIONS

■ **American Veterinary Medical Association**
https://www.avma.org

■ **Association of American Veterinary Medical Colleges**
https://www.aavmc.org

■ **American Pre-Veterinary Medical Association**
https://www.apvma.org

■ **International Council for Veterinary Assessment**
https://www.icva.net

■ **American Association of Veterinary Clinicians (AAVC)**
https://www.aavcvet.org

PERIODICALS

■ **Veterinary Practice News**
www.veterinarypracticenews.com

■ **Clinicians Brief**
http://www.cliniciansbrief.com

■ **Zoo News Digest**
http://zoonewsdigest.blogspot.com

WEBSITES

■ **A Veterinary Student**
https://vinfoundation.org/i-am
/veterinary-student

■ **Global Leadership Adventures (GLA)**
www.experiencegla.com/program
-types/wildlife-conservation